Emergency Aid Handbook

A Reference Guide

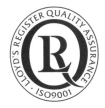

The Quality Management System is applicable to:

Central management, design and provision of training courses, training and information documents, advice and information relating to: First aid, care and associated skills/subjects; Health and safety and associated skills/subjects; Training of trainers. Provision of support services to St. John Ambulance units.

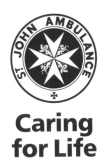

**Caring
for Life**

First published in Great Britain in 1996 by
St. John Supplies
PO Box 707B, Friend Street
London EC1V 7NE
020 7278 7888

First Edition October 1996 53/027662
Second Edition April 1997 1152/029059
Third Edition January 1999
Fourth Edition July 2001
Second Impression November 2001 53/014110
Fifth Edition July 2002 752/016142
Second Impression February 2003 53/019460
Third Impression July 2003 53/021433

ISBN: 0 900700 60 2

British Library Cataloguing in Publication Data.
A catalogue for this book is available from the British Library.

St. John Supplies Product R00158U

Printed in England by Lamport Gilbert Ltd

Contents

Page

Introduction	4
Incident Management	5
Casualty Management and Initial Assessment	7
Recovery Position	10
Rescue Breaths for Adults	13
Cardio-Pulmonary Resuscitation for Adults	16
Cardio-Pulmonary Resuscitation for Babies and Children	20
Recognition and Treatment of Choking	23
Secondary Survey	27
Recognition and Treatment of Shock	30
Recognition and Treatment of Heart Attacks	33
Recognition and Treatment of Wounds and Bleeding	36
Recognition and Treatment of Fainting	43
Recognition and Treatment of Burns	45
Recognition and Stabilisation of Fractures	50
Recognition and Treatment of Head Injuries	56
Recognition and Treatment of Soft Tissue Injuries	60
Recognition and Treatment of Asthma	63
Recognition and Treatment of Hypoglycaemia	65
Recognition and Treatment of Epileptic Seizures	67
Recognition and Treatment of a Stroke	71
The General Treatment of Poisoning	73
The Treatment of Bites and Stings	77
What Next?	84

Introduction

This book is not designed to turn you into a First Aider. It will provide you with the basic information to help you make the appropriate decisions and to provide care at the scene of an accident or sudden illness. This may prevent a casualty's condition from becoming worse or may even save someone's life.

This book will help you after you have finished your Emergency Aid course to remember the important issues that your Trainer has discussed with you. To help you find that information quickly each chapter has specific headings.

Background notes – Provide information about the condition or injury.

Recognition features – Describe the way in which the casualties will look or feel when you find them.

Aim – This short section will tell you in a few words what you will hope to achieve by providing Emergency Aid.

Actions – This section will tell you in a step-by-step manner exactly what to do.

Enjoy the course and this book. Don't forget that St. John Ambulance can provide you with additional training in an ever-growing number of First Aid and care-related courses. Contact your local County Office or Training Centre for more details.

Incident Management

Background Information

To enable you to provide safe and effective assistance at the scene of an emergency you need to work in a logical and planned manner. The first stage of this plan is Incident Management.

Imagine you are walking along a country lane. You hear a loud bang and see a bright flash behind the hedgerow. A boy has tangled his kite in overhead high voltage cables by the railway. You see two people running towards him.

- What is your first thought?
- What is your first impulse?
- What would you do?
- Is there a sequence of thoughts or actions you might consider?

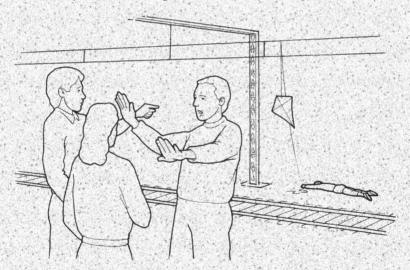

The first thing to do in any incident is to consider the **safety of yourself and others**. The last thing you want is more casualties than necessary, so look for danger to yourself and then to the casualty. Think about the scenario, you will need to keep people at least 18 metres away from the high voltage cables and contact the emergency services for medical aid and assistance.

Actions

Assess the situation

Ask yourself and others these questions:

- What has happened?
- Has anyone been hurt?
- Is there anyone hidden from view or trapped somewhere?

Make the situation safe

- Depending on the situation contact the emergency services before going near the scene.
- Try to remove or reduce any danger.
- If this is not possible remove the casualty from the danger.

Decide on what action you need to take

- Provide emergency aid to any casualties.

Get Help

- The sooner the better.
- Send a bystander to phone for an ambulance if it is required.

Tidy up

After any incident make sure that:

- Any debris is cleared away.
- Try to remove the cause of the accident if possible, or, take professional advice on repairs.
- Replenish your First Aid kit.
- We all have worries and fears after dealing with an incident, so talk to a friend or relative about your thoughts and feelings, it helps!

Casualty Management and Initial Assessment

Background Information

Once you have the incident under control you then need to think about how you are going to deal with the casualty. These simple steps will show you how to deal with any casualty.

A key principle to remember is that a person needs oxygen to survive. If the supply of oxygen is lost for more than 3 minutes, irreversible brain damage or death may occur. Oxygen is supplied to the body from the air and is transferred to the brain and other vital organs by the blood supply. The functions of being able to breathe and to pump blood around the body are essential to life.

Actions

DANGER: Don't forget to check for danger to yourself and then to the casualty. Remove any hazard that you safely can or, if absolutely necessary, move the casualty away from the danger. Remember that the emergency services are all too familiar with Good Samaritans who become seriously injured or are even killed at the scene of an accident because they forgot to look before they leapt!

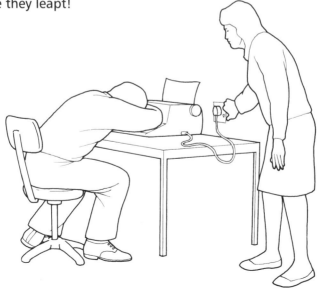

RESPONSE: Check to see if your casualty is conscious, shout a command, "Open your eyes if you can hear me!". Then give them a gentle shake, not too roughly as you might make any injuries worse. Remember, if your casualty is unconscious then they are at risk from a blocked airway, so shout for help and move quickly to the next stage.

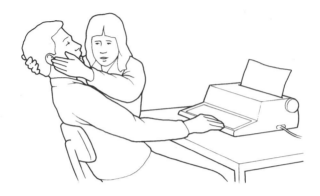

AIRWAY: Most people who die at the scene of an accident do so because they become unconscious and their airway (windpipe) becomes blocked. Place one hand on the casualty's forehead and tilt their head back. Remove any obvious obstructions from the mouth and then lift the chin with 2 fingers.

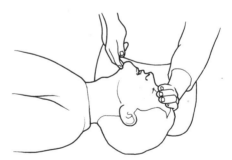

BREATHING: Once the airway has been obstructed for a period of time, then breathing will stop! Quite often, once the airway has been opened, the casualty will start breathing again. If not, then you will have to breathe for the casualty, by giving Rescue Breaths. Check for breathing by opening the airway and placing your cheek just above his mouth and nose, listen and feel for his breath for ten seconds. Look to the chest, watch for movement.

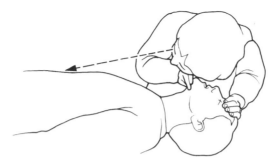

CIRCULATION: There are two ways in which circulation may affect the way we move oxygen around the body:

● The heart may stop. If it does then we need to pump the blood around the body, Cardio-Pulmonary Resuscitation (CPR). We can check for circulation by looking, listening and feeling for breathing, coughing, movement or any other signs of life.

● There may be a leak in the system – bleeding. We need to check for any leaks so that we can plug them as soon as possible.

So we can see that remembering the initial assessment and priorities of treatment is as simple as DRABC.

Danger

Response

Airway

Breathing

Circulation

The Recovery Position

Background Information

We have seen that the person who is unconscious is at risk from dying because of a blocked airway. In most cases this can be prevented by turning the casualty into the recovery position as soon as you have made sure they are breathing.

Aim

- **Maintain the casualty's airway**

Actions

Place the casualty into the recovery position using the following steps:

1 Kneel beside the casualty as closely as you can.

2 Open the airway by lifting the chin and gently tilting the head back.

3 Place the arm nearest you at right angles to the body, palm upwards.

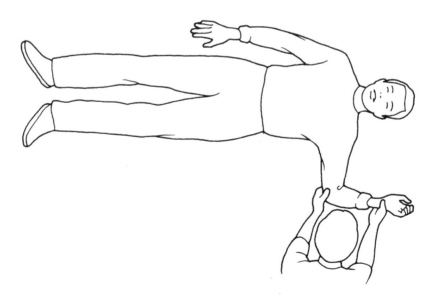

4 Bring the arm furthest away from you over the chest holding his hand palm out, and place the back of his hand against the cheek nearest you.

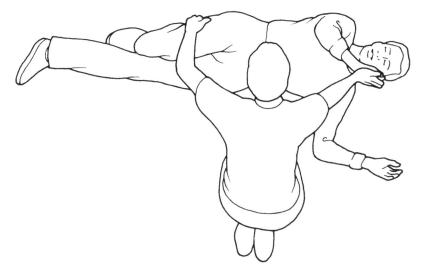

5 Using your other hand grasp the thigh furthest away from you and pull the knee up; make sure that the foot is flat on the floor.

6 Keep your hand pressed to the cheek to support the head and neck and pull his thigh towards you, so rolling the casualty onto his side.

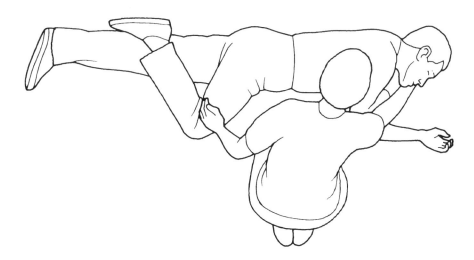

7 Bring the upper leg towards the hip so that the knee and the hip are at right angles.

8 Gently tilt the head back to keep an open airway and, if necessary, adjust the hand under the cheek to support the head. Keep the mouth pointing towards the floor.

9 If injuries allow, turn the casualty onto the other side every 30 minutes.

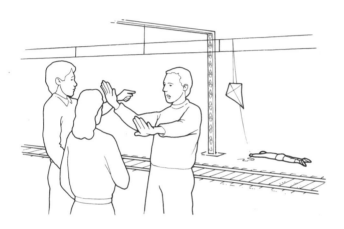

This simple move can save countless lives every year!

NOTE: If you suspect spinal injury, steady and support the head in a neutral position and open the casualty's airway by using a jaw thrust. This is where you place your hands on either side of the face, with your fingertips at the angles of the jaw, and gently lift the jaw to open the airway (taking care not to tilt the casualty's neck).

Rescue Breaths for Adults

Being faced with a casualty who has stopped breathing can be a frightening experience, but keeping a cool head and remembering a few simple steps you may be able to help prevent a tragedy.

Recognition features

✗ *Unconsciousness*

✗ *No signs of breathing*

✗ *Increasing blueness of the skin (cyanosis)*

Aim

● *Maintain a supply of oxygen to the body*

If the casualty is not breathing and there is no history of injury, drowning or choking – go for help immediately. Reassess DRAB and, if there is still no breathing, begin Rescue Breaths.

If the casualty is not breathing due to injury, drowning or choking – begin Rescue Breaths, following the sequence through Steps 1-9, and then go for help. Reassess DRAB and, if there is still no breathing, begin sequence again.

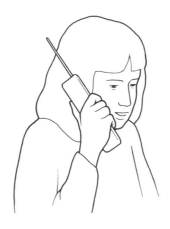

Actions

1 Ensure, as far as possible, that the casualty is flat on his back and that the airway is open.

2 Pinch the casualty's nose.

3 Take a full breath.

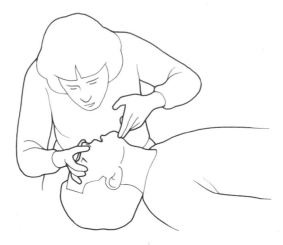

4 Place your mouth over the casualty's mouth and make a good seal.

5 Breathe into the casualty's mouth until you see the chest rise.

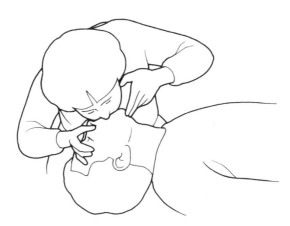

6 Remove your mouth and let their chest fall.

7 Give a second Rescue Breath, as above.

8 Check for circulation for ten seconds.

9 If circulation is present, give a further ten breaths as above.

10 Check circulation again.

11 You should aim to provide about ten breaths per minute. Don't try to get more in, you will exhaust yourself. Remember to check circulation after every ten breaths. You need to keep this up until help arrives.

If you cannot make the chest rise when you breathe into the casualty, then check that:

● The head is tilted back far enough.

● You have a good seal around the mouth.

● You have pinched the nostrils firmly enough.

● The airway is not obstructed. Look in the mouth, but don't blindly fish around with fingers if you can't see anything. You might push an obstruction further down the throat.

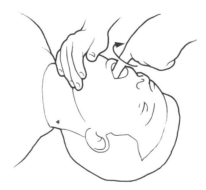

● Try giving 2 rescue breaths 5 more times.

● If you still cannot get the chest to rise, begin chest compressions immediately.

Cardio-Pulmonary Resuscitation for Adults

Background Information

Thousands of people die every year from heart attacks. Many of these deaths could be prevented if people had the basic skills of CPR.

If you find yourself dealing with a heart attack victim whose heart has stopped or a person who has been seriously injured who has a cardiac arrest, then these simple steps can save life.

Recognition features

✗ Unconsciousness

✗ No signs of breathing, coughing or movement

✗ Pupils will be open wide

✗ Very pale in appearance

✗ Increasing blueness of the skin (cyanosis)

Aim

● Maintain circulation to the casualty's vital organs

Actions

● First of all do your initial assessment. (DRABC).

● If you find that the casualty has stopped breathing go for help straight away unless there are signs of injury, drowning or choking in which case you should give 2 effective Rescue Breaths and check for circulation. If there is no circulation carry out 1 minute CPR before going for help.

When you return, reassess DRAB and if the casualty is still not breathing give two breaths and check the circulation.

1 Locate the right spot to do the chest compressions by placing your fingers on the edge of the ribs (where they meet the tummy) and run your finger up to the bottom of the breast bone. Put your middle finger on the bottom of the breast bone and your index finger next to that.

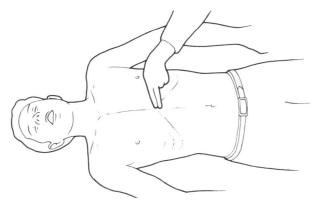

2 Now place the heel of your other hand next to your fingers, take the fingers away and place this hand on top of the one that is on the breast bone. Interlock your fingers and keep them up off the ribs.

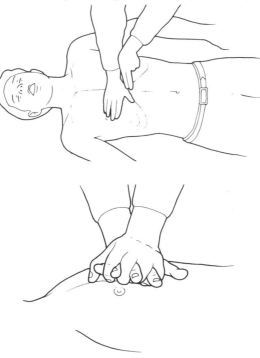

3 Now press down 4-5 cms, keeping your elbows straight, then release the pressure but do not take your hands off the chest. Repeat this 15 times then give 2 breaths.

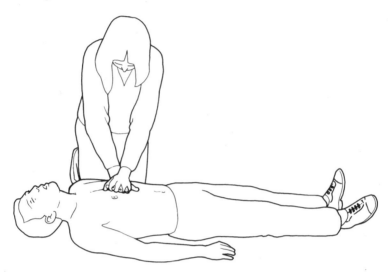

4 Continue giving 15 compressions to 2 breaths, repeating this cycle about 4 times per minute until help arrives. Don't stop to check for circulation unless you think that the casualty is improving.

It is now well understood that CPR in many cases does not restart the heart but it buys time by pumping oxygen around the body to the vital organs until professional help arrives, such as a paramedic. It is the job of the paramedic or the doctor to try and start the heart again using specialised equipment such as defibrillators and drugs. This forms part of the chain of survival:

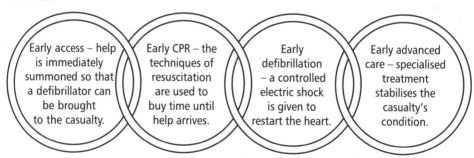

Early access – help is immediately summoned so that a defibrillator can be brought to the casualty.

Early CPR – the techniques of resuscitation are used to buy time until help arrives.

Early defibrillation – a controlled electric shock is given to restart the heart.

Early advanced care – specialised treatment stabilises the casualty's condition.

You can see that to provide the last two links in the chain you need to get help as soon as possible but if you are alone you should:

● go for help immediately if there are no signs of injury

● do 1 minute CPR before going for help if the cardiac arrest is due to injury, drowning or choking.

Also, don't forget to tell the ambulance crew about your findings and actions.

Many people are worried about giving Rescue Breaths and the dangers of HIV. Well don't! There has been no evidence to link giving Rescue Breaths and acquiring HIV. The only danger that may be present is if the casualty has facial wounds or open sores around the mouth. You can buy, very cheaply, simple plastic face shields to protect yourself in these cases.

Cardio-Pulmonary Resuscitation for Babies and Children

Background Information

Children on the whole are extremely healthy and do not suffer from the health problems that we see in adults, such as heart disease. Even so, many children each year require resuscitation because of the effects of an accident or sudden illness. This course will not teach you resuscitation skills for babies and children. You need to take a special course designed for that purpose.

St. John Ambulance runs these courses on a regular basis. Please telephone your local County office for details.

We have included here a few notes to explain the differences between performing resuscitation on adults, children and babies.

Recognition features

✗ *Unconsciousness*

✗ *No signs of breathing, coughing or movement*

✗ *Pupils will be open wide*

✗ *Very pale in appearance*

✗ *Increasing blueness of the skin (cyanosis)*

Aim

● *Maintain circulation to the casualty's vital organs*

Children aged One to Seven (inclusive)

Actions

1 Remember, begin with the initial assessment (DRABC). If there is no breathing:

2 Ensure the airway is open.

3 Pinch the nose and give two effective breaths, enough to make the chest rise and no more. Allow the chest to fall between each breath.

4 Check for circulation.

5 If there is circulation, then give twenty breaths, over a minute.

6 Call for help and, if possible, take the child with you to the phone.

7 When you have finished your call reassess DRAB, give 2 breaths, check C. If there is no change then continue with twenty breaths per minute and check the circulation after every twenty breaths.

8 If when you first check for circulation you find nothing, give five chest compressions to one breath for one minute then go for help if someone has not already done so. Again, if you can, take the child with you. *You find the right spot for chest compressions as you would for an adult but use one hand only and much lighter pressure, compress the chest about ¹/₃ of the depth of the chest.*

9 After you have made the call then reassess DRAB, give 2 breaths, check C. If there is still no circulation continue with five compressions to one breath, try to fit fifteen to twenty cycles in per minute.

Babies under One

Actions

1 Assess DRAB. If there is no breathing:

2 Ensure the airway is open.

3 Seal your mouth around the baby's mouth and nose.

4 Give two gentle but effective breaths, just enough to make the chest rise. Allow the chest to fall between each breath.

5 Check for circulation.

6 If there is circulation give twenty breaths over a minute, then go for help taking baby with you.

7 If there is no circulation start chest compressions. *To find the right spot for compressions draw an imaginary line between the nipples and then place two fingers on the breast bone one finger's width below that line. You need to press very gently, about $^1/_3$ of the depth of the chest.*

8 Give five compressions and one breath and continue that for a minute before going for help.

9 After you have made your call, reassess DRAB, give 2 breaths, check C and continue with resuscitation as required until help arrives.

Remember to tell the ambulance crew about your actions and findings.

Recognition and Treatment of Choking

Background Information

Every year a number of people choke to death on food or other objects placed in the mouth. Thankfully most choking incidents are fairly minor, even so these are frightening for the casualty as well as for the person looking after them.

Recognition features

✗ Difficulty in breathing or speaking

✗ Grasping at the neck

✗ Pointing to mouth and throat

✗ Purple/Red colour around the face and neck

✗ Blueness to lips

Aim

● Remove the obstruction and allow the casualty to breathe normally

Actions

1 Reassure the casualty, bend him forward with his head lower than his chest and encourage him to cough.

2 If the casualty stops coughing or becomes very weak slap up to five times between the shoulder blades. See if you can now remove the obstruction.

3 If this is unsuccessful, try up to five abdominal thrusts. Stand behind the casualty, link your hands below his rib cage, then pull sharply, inward and upwards.

4 If this is unsuccessful dial 999 for an ambulance.

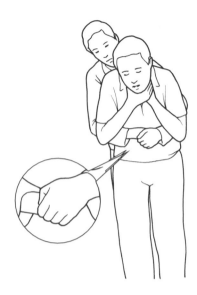

5 Keep repeating the cycle of back slaps and abdominal thrusts until the airway is clear or until help arrives.

6 If the casualty becomes unconscious, check the breathing. If they have stopped breathing, take the following steps:

7 Start Rescue Breaths, it may be possible to ventilate the casualty if the obstruction is only partial. Try up to 5 breaths.

8 If you are unable to get the breaths into the casualty then begin chest compressions immediately.

9 If you <u>are</u> able to ventilate the casualty, check for circulation and continue breaths or CPR as required.

10 If the casualty is breathing, place him in the recovery position and call for an ambulance if you have not already done so.

The treatment for babies and children is slightly different. Let's review these differences.

Recognition features

✗ *The child's face may go red at first*

✗ *The skin is likely to become paler, with a bluish tint*

✗ *They will be fighting for breath*

Aim

● *Remove the obstruction and allow the casualty to breathe normally*

Look in the mouth and try to remove any visible object with a finger. **DO NOT** touch the back of the throat with your fingers; in a young child this is very soft and may swell or bleed, further blocking the airway.

DO NOT probe blindly into the mouth – you may push the object further into the airway.

If the baby or child is not breathing then start Rescue Breaths immediately – it may be possible to ventilate the baby or child if the obstruction is only partial.

Child (aged one to seven years)

Actions

1 Encourage the child to cough if possible.

2 If the child stops coughing or becomes very weak, bend the child forwards, so that the head is lower then the chest and give up to five firm slaps between the shoulder blades. Check the mouth.

3 If this does not work, stand or kneel behind the child and give up to 5 chest thrusts. Use the same hand position as you use for chest compressions in resuscitation but with two hands pull more sharply at a rate of about 1 every 3 seconds. Check the mouth again.

4 If this does not work, give abdominal thrusts; stand behind the child, put your arms around their waist and link your hands together. Give a sharp pull inwards and upwards below the child's ribs. Repeat up to 5 times. Check the mouth again.

5 If this still has not cleared the airway, dial 999 for an ambulance. Continue repeating the sequence of back slaps, chest thrusts, abdominal thrusts until help arrives or the airway is clear. If breathing stops at any time, start Rescue Breaths.

Babies (under 1 year)

Actions

1 Lay the baby along your forearm or thigh with the face down and the head low and supported.

2 Give up to 5 firm slaps between the shoulder blades. Check the mouth.

3 If this does not work, turn the baby on its back along your thigh head down. Give up to 5 chest thrusts. Use the same technique and finger position as you use for chest compressions in resuscitation but press more sharply at a rate of about 1 every 3 seconds. Check the mouth again.

4 If this does not clear the obstruction repeat the sequence of back slaps and chest thrusts three times then take the baby with you to call for help.

5 Continue repeating the sequence until help arrives.

DO NOT USE ABDOMINAL THRUSTS ON A BABY UNDER 1 YEAR

Finally, remember when dealing with choking, if the obstruction is not cleared straight away call for urgent assistance. It is better for an ambulance to arrive to find a pink and screaming child than a tragedy.

Secondary Survey

Background Information

Once you have provided the initial emergency treatment for the casualty, the next step is to look for further clues to find out what is wrong with the person.

This process of systematically examining the person is called the Secondary survey.

As with all First Aid procedures we can follow a simple routine. To carry out the survey you will need to use both your hands to examine the person and compare and contrast the opposite sides of the body. Look carefully at the casualty and the situation he is in. Also, don't forget to ask the casualty and onlookers questions and listen carefully to any answers. Remember that your sense of smell may also provide you with clues, for example chemical smells, alcohol, etc.

Let's look at the procedure in detail. Remember that you will have carried out your initial assessment (Primary survey) already.

Aim

- *Using a systematic approach, identify any other injuries or problems the casualty may have.*

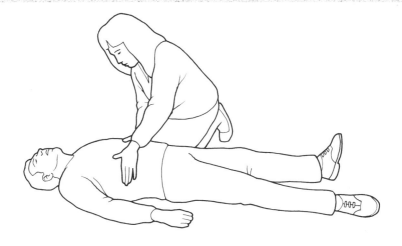

Actions

Remember if the casualty is unconscious he may vomit and obstruct his airway without you being aware. Therefore it may be advantageous to place the casualty in the recovery position prior to starting the Secondary survey.

1 Run your hands over the person's scalp looking for bleeding, swelling or indentation. Try not to move the head and neck at this point.

2 Look into each ear for any blood or fluid.

3 Open the eyes and check the pupils for size and reaction to light. The pupils should be equal, a normal size and react equally.

4 Check the nose for blood or fluid.

5 Check the rate and depth of breathing; also note any unusual odour in the breath.

6 Check in the mouth for anything that may be blocking the airway. DO NOT remove dentures unless they are loose. Also check for any wounds.

7 Look at the face for any wounds or irregularity to the natural lines.

8 Note the colour and temperature of the skin.

9 Loosen the clothing around the neck; look for any wounds or swelling to the neck tissues. Also look for signs of the person being a neck breather. There may be a stoma or hole in the front of the neck below the area of the Adam's apple.

10 Look for a "medic alert" type necklace and talisman.

11 Check the carotid pulse and make a note of the rate, rhythm and strength.

12 Gently place your hands under the neck without causing movement and carefully feel the bones of the neck and the base of the skull, looking for any irregularity or swelling.

13 Move your hands down the chest again feeling for swelling, irregularity or wounds. If the casualty is conscious then ask him to take a deep breath and assess the chest for equal and even movements.

14 Place your hands at the top of the chest and gently move them along the shoulders to check for swelling and irregularity.

15 Check each arm in turn for any wounds or irregularity. If the casualty is conscious then ask him to bend and straighten fingers and elbows. Check for information bracelet.

16 Check each hand and finger for injury.

17 Without causing undue movement place your hands under the small of the back and gently feel along the bones of the back for swelling and irregularity.

18 Look at the abdomen for wounds or bruising, then place a hand on the casualty's abdomen and press down gently, looking for tenderness and rigidity.

19 Place your hands on either side of the hips and gently rock the pelvis, noting any difference or irregularity in motion. Make a note of any sign of incontinence or bleeding from the genital or anal areas.

20 Examine each leg in turn for wounds and swelling. If the casualty is conscious ask him to move each joint in turn.

21 Check each foot and the ankle for swelling irregularity and movement.

When you have completed the survey treat any problems you may have found. Also, it will be useful to note down any abnormalities you may have found so that this information can be passed to the emergency services.

Recognition and Treatment of Shock

Background Information

The circulation system of the body distributes blood to all parts of the body. This allows oxygen and nutrients to reach individual cells (the smallest living parts of the body). When injury or sudden illness affects this system and vital cells such as those in the brain, heart and lungs no longer receive a reasonable blood supply then the condition known as shock sets in. Shock, or the cause of it, if not treated promptly by the person with First Aid knowledge can be fatal.

Recognition features

X Pale, ashen, cold, clammy skin

X Rapid pulse, becoming weaker as time progresses

X Rapid shallow breathing

X Nausea and possibly vomiting

X The casualty will feel weak and giddy and complain of thirst

X The casualty may be restless and anxious, possibly aggressive

X The casualty may yawn or gasp for air

X Decreasing consciousness

Aims

● Treat any obvious cause

● Increase the blood supply to the brain, heart and lungs

● Get urgent medical help

Actions

1 Treat the cause of shock.

2 If injuries allow, lay the casualty down, keep the head low (don't use pillows) and raise the legs gently. This will help to keep blood in the vital areas such as the brain.

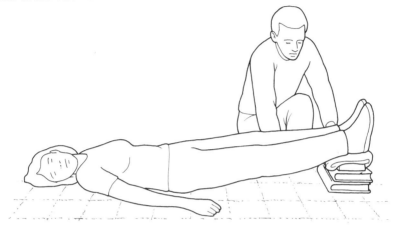

3 Try to keep her as still and quiet as possible. Give plenty of reassurance.

4 Loosen tight clothing around the neck, chest and waist.

5 Try if possible to get a blanket under the casualty and cover her with a blanket. Don't be tempted to pile blankets or coats on to the casualty; this may be harmful.

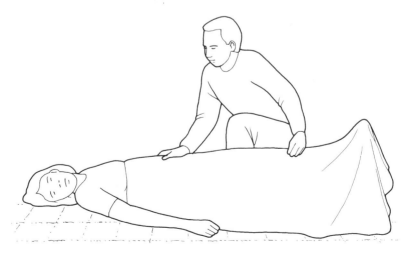

31

6 Dial 999 for an ambulance.

7 Do not give anything to eat or drink or let her smoke. If the casualty complains of thirst, moisten the lips.

8 Keep a check on her breathing, pulse and level of consciousness; you may need to resuscitate her.

9 If she becomes unconscious then put her in the recovery position.

10 Make notes for the ambulance crew on your findings and actions.

Recognition and Treatment of Heart Attacks

Background Information

Unfortunately heart attacks are becoming more common, so people with First Aid knowledge are more and more likely to have to deal with them. Also the age of the person liable to have a heart attack is becoming lower.

Recognition features

✗ *Persistent crushing, vice-like pain in the centre of the chest*

✗ *The pain may spread down into the left arm and up into the neck and jaw*

✗ *The pain does not go away with rest; it may even occur at rest*

✗ *There may be pain or discomfort in the abdomen, like indigestion*

✗ *The casualty may be breathless*

✗ *The skin will look "ashen" with a blueness to lips*

✗ *The pulse will be rapid, becoming weaker and may be irregular in its rhythm*

✗ *The casualty may feel faint or giddy*

✗ *There may be an overwhelming feeling of terror*

✗ *The casualty may collapse, with no breathing and no circulation, without warning*

Aims

● *Cut down on the workload of the heart*

● *Get urgent medical help*

Actions

1 Make the casualty as comfortable as possible by putting him into a half sitting position. Make sure that his head and shoulders are supported and if possible put a coat or blanket under the knees to provide additional support. This will help their breathing.

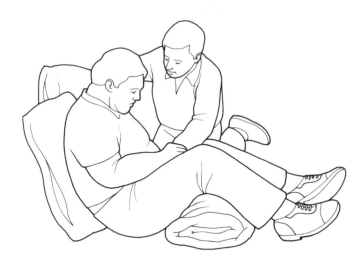

2 Call for an ambulance and tell the control that you suspect that the person is having a heart attack. If you are able to, and if the casualty wishes, call his own doctor as well.

3 Cover the person with a blanket; he may well be cold due to shock.

4 If the casualty is conscious then give him an Aspirin tablet if you have one available and tell him to chew it slowly. This can prevent the heart from being damaged too much.

5 Keep a close eye on the casualty's breathing as it may stop at any time. Be prepared to resuscitate.

6 If the casualty becomes unconscious then place him in the recovery position.

7 Make a note of all you do and find, to inform the ambulance service.

Another condition that will give similar recognition features is Angina. This often comes on with exercise and will normally go away with rest. The casualty may have her own medication as a spray or a tablet to put under the tongue.

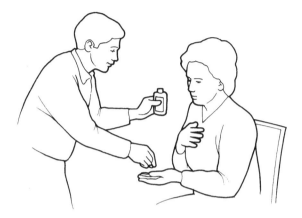

Let the casualty take this and rest. If the pain persists then treat as a heart attack and dial 999 for an ambulance.

35

Recognition and Treatment of Wounds and Bleeding

Background Information

Any break in the surface of the skin or body surfaces is termed as a wound. Wounds can be described as open or closed.

Open wounds – Most open wounds are the everyday cuts and grazes, but some may be more serious and involve severe bleeding.

Closed wounds – The closed wound which a person with First Aid knowledge will most commonly deal is a simple bruise. Bruising can be severe if there is underlying injury such as fracture.

The body will lose blood and other body fluids from a wound and, if the wound is open, germs may enter. This may lead to infection. As always the person with First Aid knowledge has to consider her own safety. Blood and other body fluids can carry viruses such as HIV and Hepatitis B. If possible, before carrying out any First Aid you should put on disposable gloves, not the polythene type but good quality latex. Make it a practice to keep sore or open areas covered with waterproof dressings. If your skin does come into contact with a large quantity of blood or you are splashed in the eyes or mouth, or if you prick or cut your own skin, then urgently seek advice from your own doctor.

Let us deal with each type of wound in turn. In all cases remember your initial assessment, DRABC, and deal with each priority in turn.

Aims

- *Control the blood loss*
- *Treat for shock*
- *Prevent infection*
- *Where appropriate, arrange removal to hospital*

Minor Bleeding

Actions

If it is a small cut then encourage the wound to bleed for a few minutes (this will allow the wound to clean itself). Put on disposable gloves (if available) then apply direct pressure for up to ten minutes to stop the bleeding. If the area around the wound is dirty then clean it with fresh water and gently dry the area. Cover with a sterile dressing such as a plaster but avoid using cotton wool or lint as the fibres stick to the wound. If there is grit sticking to a graze that will not come out with simple washing, then contact your own doctor for advice.

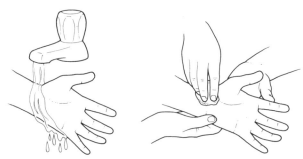

Major Bleeding

Actions

1. Put on disposable gloves if available.

2. Expose the wound being careful of any sharp objects.

3. Apply direct pressure to the wound with your fingers or palm of your hand, if there is no obvious embedded object.

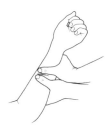

4 If there is an embedded object, apply the pressure around the sides of the wound (See point 10).

5 Use a clean pad or sterile dressing, if you have one, and raise the limb.

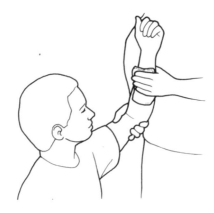

6 Lay the casualty down keeping the limb raised.

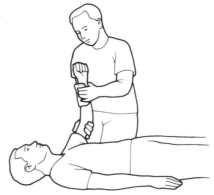

7 Treat for shock.

8 Keep the pressure on the wound for ten minutes.

9 When the bleeding is controlled, leave any original pad in place, apply a sterile dressing and bandage. Do not tie the bandage too tightly as you will cut off the circulation to the area beyond the wound.

10 If blood starts to seep though the dressing, do not remove it; put another dressing over the top and secure.

11 If blood continues to come through the second dressing, remove both dressings and re-apply a new dressing.

12 If there is an object embedded in the wound follow these steps to dress the wound:

- Place a sterile dressing lightly over the wound.

- Place padding around the dressing to build up to a point higher than the embedded object.

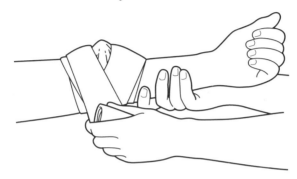

- If you cannot build up the padding high enough, bandage carefully around the object.

- Bandage lightly over the ends of the pads taking care not to put pressure on to the object below.

13 Dial 999 for an ambulance. Keep a check on breathing and pulse and also keep a check on the circulation beyond the bandage. If it is too tight then the area beyond the wound will be cold and pale and the casualty may complain of pins and needles.

14 Make a report to the ambulance crew of your findings and actions.

Bleeding from the Scalp

Background Information

Head wounds bleed very freely because the scalp has a very good blood supply and the skin and underlying tissues are stretched. This causes head wounds to gape, therefore increasing the bleeding. The person with First Aid knowledge needs to remember that an injury to the head may have also caused damage to the skull or neck. Anyone with a serious head wound or who has lost consciousness for more than three minutes due to a head injury needs to be seen by a doctor.

Actions

1 Put on disposable gloves if available.

2 If possible try to replace any displaced skin flaps.

3 Apply direct pressure with the palm of your hand, using a sterile or clean pad.

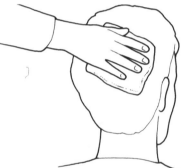

4 Do not use your fingers as this might put pressure on an underlying fracture.

5 Apply firm, direct pressure and secure the pad with a roller bandage.

6 If the casualty is conscious then lay him down keeping the head and shoulders slightly raised.

7 If he is unconscious then place him in the recovery position.

8 Arrange to get the casualty to hospital, by ambulance if the wound is serious, or if he has been unconscious.

9 Make a report to the ambulance crew or hospital staff of your findings and actions.

Nose Bleeds

Background Information

Nose bleeds are a very common problem. The most common causes are picking or scratching the internal surface, a direct blow or sneezing. There are some medical conditions that will cause nose bleeds, but regardless of the cause the treatment is the same.

Actions

1 Sit the casualty down and ensure that her head is tipped well forward. This ensures an open airway and also prevents blood from trickling down the throat causing the casualty to vomit.

2 Tell her to breathe through her mouth and to pinch the soft part of her nose just below the bridge for ten minutes.

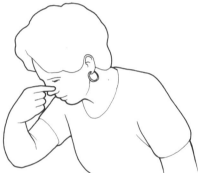

3 Tell her to try not to spit, talk, cough, swallow or sniff as this may disturb any clots. Try to provide tissues to mop up any dribble.

4 After ten minutes tell her to release the pressure. If it is still bleeding then tell her to pinch for another ten minutes.

5 If a nose bleed lasts for more than thirty minutes then the casualty must be seen by a doctor. Transport the casualty in the treatment position.

6 Once the bleeding has been stopped and with the casualty still leaning forward, gently clean around the area with luke warm water. Also offer a mouth wash.

7 Advise her to rest for a few hours to prevent the clot being disturbed, and to avoid blowing the nose or picking at any clots.

Bruising

Background Information

Bruising is a form of internal bleeding. Bruises are nearly always caused by a direct blow or injury to the area. Most develop slowly and do not require First Aid treatment. The type of bruise that you, as the person with First Aid knowledge, will have to deal with are the bruises that appear quickly with accompanying swelling. This type of bruising may indicate deeper injury.

Aims

- **Reduce the blood supply to the area**
- **Reduce the swelling, bruising and pain**

Actions

1 If necessary lay the casualty down and raise the injured part into a comfortable position. If you are worried there might be a fracture or other injuries, then seek medical advice or call for an ambulance.

2 Apply a cold compress to the area for about five minutes. If necessary bandage the compress in place. Do not use a crepe-type bandage, you may cut off the circulation to the area beyond the injury. If you use ice or frozen goods for the compress ensure that these are wrapped in a tea towel or similar cloth before applying to the skin and keep checking the area. You may cause ice burns if you don't.

3 If you send the casualty to hospital then make a report of your findings and actions.

Recognition and Treatment of Fainting

Background Information

Fainting is a reasonably common and simple condition for the person with First Aid knowledge to deal with. It occurs because the brain, for a very short period of time, does not receive an adequate blood supply. This may be due to standing around for a long period of time or a sudden shock. Fainting may also occur in the early stages of pregnancy.

Recognition features

✖ *Collapse and loss of consciousness*

✖ *Pale, cold, clammy skin*

✖ *Slow pulse, this will increase as the casualty recovers*

Aim

● *Improve the blood supply to the brain and reassure the casualty*

Actions

1 Lay the casualty down and gently raise and support the legs.

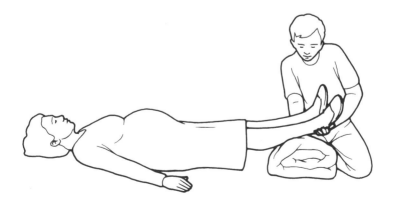

2 Provide a source of fresh air by opening a door or window.

3 As the casualty recovers plenty of reassurance will be required.

4 Sit him up slowly: if he sits up too quickly then he may faint again. If he does feel faint then lay him down again.

5 If the casualty does not regain consciousness quickly then reassess RABC, place in the recovery position and call for an ambulance.

Often someone will feel faint but not actually faint. Treat as if they have fainted.

Recognition and Treatment of Burns

Background Information

The person with First Aid knowledge may find that burns are amongst the most distressing type of injury to deal with due to the pain the casualty suffers.

Both burns and scalds are commonly caused by heat, burns by dry heat, such as fire; and scalds by moist heat, such as steam. Chemicals can also cause burns by the release of heat when contact is made with tissue. Other causes of burns may be friction, electricity and intense cold. Because of the different ways in which burns may occur you may hear them being referred to as thermal injuries. The possiblity of non-accidental injury should be considered.

Recognition features

All thermal injuries are described as having three depths:

X **Superficial**
   - X **Redness**
   - X **Tenderness**
   - X **Swelling**

X **Partial Thickness**
   - X **Redness**
   - X **Tenderness**
   - X **Swelling**
   - X **Raw appearance**
   - X **Blistering**

X **Full Thickness**
   - X **Pale and waxy**
   - X **Charred tissue**
   - X **N.B. the areas surrounding a full thickness burn may have partial thickness and superficial burns**

Although it is important for the person with First Aid knowledge to remember the depth of burns, it is more important to remember that it is the extent not the depth that is the danger. A person is more likely to suffer serious consequences from superficial burns covering 30% of the body than a full thickness burn covering 15%. As a guide, partial thickness burns greater in size than the palm of the casualty's hand and superficial burns greater than five times the palm area should receive medical aid. Other burns that need hospital attention are: full thickness burns; burns to the hands, face, feet or genital area; any burn that extends right around an arm or leg; any burn to a child or elderly person.

Minor Burns and Scalds

Aims
- *Stop the burning*
- *Relieve pain and swelling*
- *Minimise the risk of infection*

Actions

1 Flood the injured area in running cold water for ten minutes (if running water is not available then any cold harmless fluid will do), until the pain subsides.

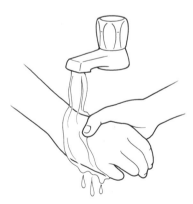

2 Gently remove anything of a constrictive nature, such as rings and watches, from the affected area.

3 Cover the area with a sterile dressing. A polythene bag or "cling" film will make an adequate temporary dressing. Clean towels will also make a suitable dressing.

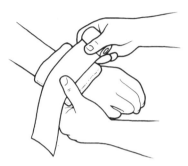

Do not use fluffy materials or adhesive dressing.

Do not burst any blisters.

Do not apply any creams, lotions or fats to the injury.

Severe Burns

Severe burns and scalds will pose a greater problem to the person with First Aid knowledge. The circumstances surrounding the incident may give you clues to the extent and depth of the burns.

Aims

- *Stop the burning and relieve pain*
- *Resuscitate, if required*
- *Treat other injuries sustained in the incident*
- *Minimise the risk of infection*
- *Contact the ambulance service urgently*

Actions

1 Lay the casualty down trying to protect the burned area from contact with the ground.

2 Start to cool the burnt area with copious amounts of cold liquid. The cooling must continue for ten minutes. This must not delay the transfer to hospital. (Be aware that overcooling the casualty may carry the risk of causing hypothermia.)

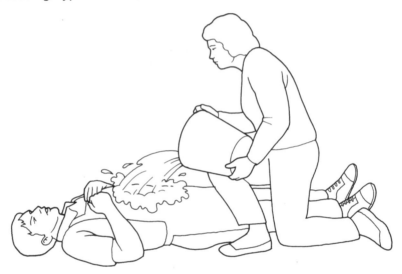

3 Whilst cooling the burn monitor the casualty closely.

4 Remove anything of a constrictive nature before swelling occurs. Also remove any smouldering clothing, but do not remove anything sticking to the burned area as this may also damage surrounding tissue.

Burns to Mouth and Throat

Burns and scalds occurring in this area can be a life-threatening problem. Rapid swelling can occur in the soft tissues of the throat leading to breathing difficulties.

Recognition features

X *Soot around the mouth and nose*

X *Singed nasal hairs*

X *Burns to mouth and nose*

X *Hoarseness of the voice*

X *Difficulty in breathing*

Aim

● *Obtain urgent medical aid*

Actions

1 Contact the ambulance service as soon as possible and say that the casualty is suffering from burns to the airway.

2 Ensure the casualty has an adequate air supply; loosen tight clothing around the neck.

3 If the casualty is conscious give sips of cold water.

4 If the casualty shows signs of losing consciousness then place him in the recovery position.

5 Be prepared to resuscitate.

Recognition and Stabilisation of Fractures

Background Information

A fracture is a break or a crack in a bone. Bone is not a brittle substance in normal healthy people, but is a tough, resilient living tissue. A lot of force is needed to damage this substance, but in the older person or the person suffering with a disease that affects bone, much less force is required.

When bone breaks it may do so in several ways:
- Chip or crack
- Clean break through the bone
- Twist or split
- Shatter or crumble

When a bone breaks, surrounding tissue will also be damaged. The degree of damage will be dependent upon the force involved in the injury. In a simple fracture the damage to surrounding tissue may be minimal but it is possible that the ends of the bone may protrude through the skin. In very severe fractures the bone ends may damage organs or major blood vessels.

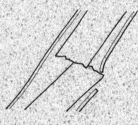 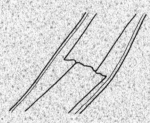

Recognition features

✗ *History of a recent blow or fall*

✗ *Sound of snapping from the injury site*

✗ *Difficulty in moving the limb*

✗ *Severe pain and tenderness over the site of the injury*

✗ *Distortion or swelling*

✗ *Bruising*

✗ *Signs of shock if the injury is severe*

The treatment for closed fractures is a very simple process known as steady and support.

Aims

● *Prevent movement at the site of injury*

● *Arrange transfer to medical aid maintaining comfortable support*

Actions

1 Warn the casualty to keep still.

2 If the injury is in the upper limb then the casualty is likely to be supporting the injured limb in the most comfortable position. It is probable there is no more that you can do.

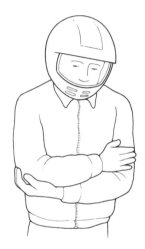

3 If the injury is in the lower limb, apply support with your hands above and below the injury.

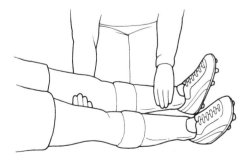

51

4 If the jaw is injured, place a soft pad under the jaw and allow the casualty to support it themselves. Sit them with the head tilted forwards.

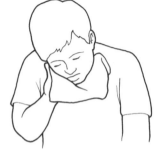

5 If the ribs have been involved, sit the casualty down in the most comfortable position for them and ask them to support the arm on the injured side.

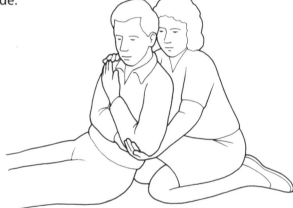

6 If the pelvis has been injured then place a rolled coat or blanket under the knees.

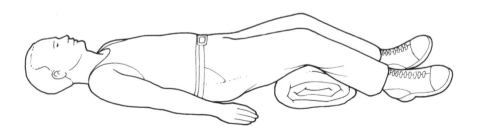

7 If you are worried that the casualty may have sustained an injury to the neck or spine then support the head and neck in the position found and get a bystander to place rolled coats or blankets around the neck and shoulders.

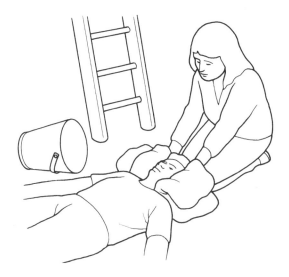

8 Treat for shock; remember, DO NOT give the casualty anything to eat or drink.

Many people are worried about moving an unconscious casualty with fractures into the recovery position. A person is more likely to die or suffer lasting disability from an obstructed airway than from a fracture. However, if you suspect spinal injury, steady and support the head in a neutral position and open the casualty's airway by using a jaw thrust. This is where you place your hands on either side of the face with your fingertips at the angles of the jaw and gently lift the jaw to open the airway, taking care not to tilt the casualty's neck.

Open Fractures

Background Information

An open fracture has the same recognition features as already described with the addition of a wound. Bone may or may not protrude through the skin.

The treatment of open fractures is much the same as that of a closed fracture.

Aims

- **Prevent blood loss, infection and movement at the site of the fracture**
- **Arrange transfer to medical aid maintaining comfortable support**

Actions

1 Warn the casualty to keep still.

2 Put on disposable gloves if available.

3 Control any bleeding from the fracture site by applying pressure to the sides of the wound.

4 Cover the wound with a sterile dressing and place padding on either side of bone if protruding.

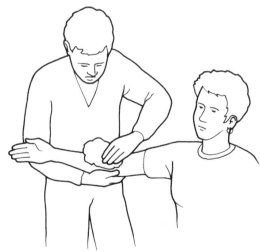

4 Secure the dressing and the padding with a bandage.

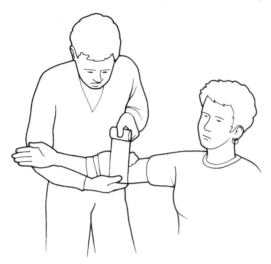

5 Steady and support as described previously.

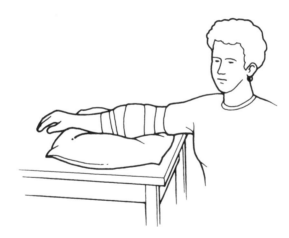

Recognition and Treatment of Head Injuries

Background Information

Although head injuries can be life threatening, thankfully most are comparatively minor, however, medical advice should always be sought. The person with First Aid knowledge must always remember that any condition that causes an altered level of consciousness may mask other injuries. Also, remember that the head injury may have been caused by the person losing consciousness for another reason, e.g. epilepsy.

Head injuries can be divided into three main types
- Concussion
- Compression
- Skull fracture

Concussion

Background Information

Let's look at concussion first. The brain is free to move a little within the skull. If the head receives a violent blow the brain can be shaken like a jelly on a plate. This can cause the person to lose consciousness. In concussion this is brief.

Recognition features
X *History of a blow to the head*
X *Brief loss of consciousness*
X *Dizziness and nausea on recovery*
X *Loss of memory of events immediately preceding the event*
X *Generalised headache*

Aims
- *Ensure that the casualty recovers fully and safely*
- *Seek medical advice if required*

Actions

1 If the casualty is unconscious but breathing, maintain an open airway.

2 Monitor levels of consciousness as well as breathing and pulse.

3 If the casualty loses consciousness for more than a few seconds then dial 999 for an ambulance.

4 When the casualty recovers, maintain a close watch for any sudden deterioration.

5 Ensure that the casualty is looked after by a responsible person. He should not continue to play sport or other such activities until he has been seen by a doctor.

6 Anyone who has suffered a blow to the head, causing even brief loss of consciousness, should be seen by a doctor.

7 All unconscious casualties with head injuries should also be treated for neck injury.

Compression

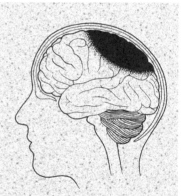

Background Information

Compression is a much more serious condition. This is where bleeding or swelling causes pressure to be put on the brain leading to a life threatening deterioration in the casualty.

Recognition features

✗ *History of a recent head injury (minutes to days)*

✗ *Apparent full recovery*

✗ *Deterioration accompanied by confusion and disorientation*

✗ *Intense headache*

✗ *Slow noisy breathing*

✗ *Slow strong pulse*

✗ *Unequal pupils*

✗ *Hot flushed appearance*

✗ *Weakness or paralysis down one side of the body*

Aim

● *Obtain urgent medical aid*

Actions

1 If the casualty is unconscious but breathing use a jaw thrust to maintain the airway.

2 Monitor breathing, pulse and levels of consciousness.

Skull Fractures

Background Information

Skull fractures may be accompanied by concussion or compression. But, in certain circumstances the casualty may not have a history of loss of consciousness following a head injury but still have a serious skull fracture.

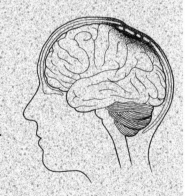

The skull may also be fractured when someone falls from a height and lands heavily on their feet causing a shock wave to travel up the spine and damage the skull.

Whenever someone sustains a head injury or a heavy fall on to their feet the person with First Aid knowledge must consider the possibility of a skull fracture.

Recognition features

✗ History of head injury or fall

✗ Wound or bruise to the head

✗ "Boggy" area or "dent" in the scalp

✗ Decreased level of consciousness

✗ Clear or blood stained fluid leaking from the nose or ears

✗ Blood in the white of the eye

✗ Distortion of head or face

Aims

● Maintenance of an open airway

● Obtain urgent medical aid

Actions

1 If the casualty is unconscious but breathing then use a jaw thrust to maintain airway and monitor the depth of unconsciousness, breathing and pulse.

2 If the casualty is conscious, lie him down. Do not let him turn his head.

3 If there is any discharge from the ear, cover with a sterile dressing or clean pad. Secure this with a light bandage. Do not plug the ear.

4 Control any bleeding from the scalp.

5 Dial 999 for an ambulance.

There is one other aspect of dealing with head injuries that the person with First Aid knowledge must remember. Any injury severe enough to cause loss of consciousness can cause injury to the neck. When dealing with any head injury you must remember to keep all movement to a minimum. Where movement is inevitable then support the head and neck as much as possible.

Recognition and Treatment of Soft Tissue Injuries

Background Information

Injuries to soft tissues can normally be divided into two main groups:

Strain: This is an injury to the muscle or tendon. A tendon is a band of tough fibrous material that connects muscle to bone.

Sprain: This is an injury to a ligament. A ligament is a band of tough fibrous tissue that provides support to joints.

Strains are painful injuries that can occur anywhere in the body and normally occur when a muscle is used suddenly and without "warming up", such as in sports injuries. Sprains, on the other hand, will always occur over a joint and be the result of sudden twisting or stretching of the joint. It may be difficult to tell the difference between a sprain and a fracture.

Recognition features

✖ *The recognition features for soft tissue injuries are much the same as for fractures. If there is any doubt as to whether the injury is a fracture or soft tissue injury, treat as a fracture.*

Aims

● *To reduce pain and swelling*

● *To obtain medical aid if required*

Actions

1 Sit or lay the casualty down.

2 Rest, steady and support the injured area. If the injury is to a limb then elevate it.

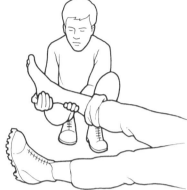

3 If the injury is recent, apply an ice pack or cold compress to the area. N.B. If you use ice then ensure that it is wrapped in a towel or similar wrap, as ice against the skin will cause a burn.

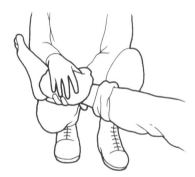

4 If the injury is to a limb, cover the ice pack in a layer of padding and then bandage securely into place.

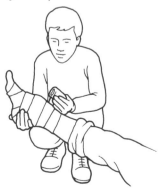

5 Keep the limb elevated and check every ten minutes that the bandage is not too tight. A tight bandage will cause increased pain and swelling, tingling beyond the bandage and discoloration of the skin.

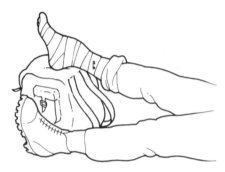

6 If the casualty does not respond to the treatment or you are unsure about the severity of the injury, then send the casualty to hospital.

The treatment for soft tissue injury can be summed up as:

Rest.

Ice.

Compression.

Elevation.

Recognition and Treatment of Asthma

Background Information

Asthma is becoming more and more prevalent every year, affecting both adults and children. It is a distressing condition that causes the small passages of the airway to constrict due to spasm. These tissues also secrete a thick and sticky mucous causing further difficulties in breathing.

An asthma attack may be triggered by many things. Common trigger factors include air pollution, cigarette smoke, pollen, dust and nervous tension.

The majority of sufferers will know how best to deal with the attack. Most asthmatics carry medication in the form of an inhaler or "puffer". This will help to alleviate the symptoms of an attack in most cases.

Despite the advances in research and the fact that most sufferers carry their medication with them, a percentage of sufferers of all ages will die each year from severe asthma attacks. Be prepared for a sudden deterioration in the person suffering from asthma.

Recognition features

✗ *Difficulty in breathing, particularly breathing out*

✗ *A wheeze may be noted when the person breathes out*

✗ *Distress and anxiety*

✗ *In a severe case the person may have great difficulty in talking*

✗ *Blueness of the lips may be present*

✗ *The casualty may have a rapid pulse*

✗ *N.B. If the last three features are present then treat as an emergency and dial 999 for an ambulance urgently*

Aims

● *Ease the casualty's breathing*

● *Arrange medical aid if required*

Actions

1 Reassure the casualty.

2 Help the casualty to sit in a comfortable position. This will probably be leaning slightly forward, supporting themselves on a table, etc.

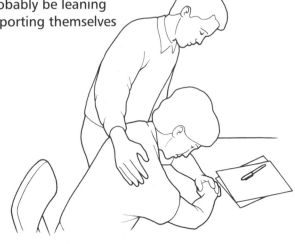

3 Ensure a supply of fresh air. Open a window if possible, providing the trigger factor is not outside air pollution such as pollen.

4 The casualty may find that a fan will help.

5 Allow the casualty to take their own medication.

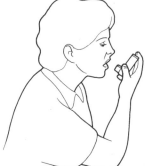

6 If the casualty responds to their medication and rest then nothing more need be done except to encourage the casualty to discuss the attack with her doctor or specialist nurse.

7 If the inhaler has no effect after five minutes or breathlessness makes it difficult for the casualty to talk, they become exhausted or their condition deteriorates, call 999 urgently.

8 Be prepared to deal with a collapsed person.

Recognition and Treatment of Hypoglycaemia

Background Information

Hypoglycaemia means low blood sugar. It is generally only seen in diabetics, but it may occur as a complication of other conditions.

Diabetics are normally prepared for the onset of low blood sugar. The most common cause for this is too little carbohydrate being taken to offset their normal dose of insulin. Exercise will increase the speed of onset of this condition.

Recognition features

✗ A history of diabetes
   ✗ May be carrying a card or other "ID"
   ✗ May be carrying insulin

✗ The casualty may recognise the onset of a "hypo"
   ✗ Weakness, faintness or hunger
   ✗ Palpitations and muscle tremors
   ✗ Confused or aggressive behaviour
   ✗ Profuse sweating
   ✗ Pale and cold to touch
   ✗ Strong bounding pulse
   ✗ Shallow breathing
   ✗ Deteriorating level of consciousness

Aims

● If the casualty is conscious, the sugar level should be raised as quickly as possible

● If the casualty is unconscious then gain medical aid as quickly as possible

Actions

1 Carry out your initial assessment.

2 If the casualty is unconscious but breathing turn him into the recovery position.

3 Dial 999 for an ambulance.

4 Be prepared to resuscitate if necessary.

5 If the casualty is conscious, help him to sit down.

6 Give a sugary drink or sugary food, such as chocolate or glucose tablets.

7 If the condition improves give more food or drink and allow the casualty to rest until fully recovered.

8 Advise the casualty to discuss this episode with his doctor.

9 If the condition does not improve rapidly then call for an ambulance.

Recognition and Treatment of Epileptic Seizures

Background Information

The condition known as epilepsy is far more common than people realise. With modern treatments most people with epilepsy live almost completely normal lives and very rarely suffer from any form of seizures. The seizures are caused by a disturbance in the electrical activity of the brain leading to a variety of symptoms.

Epileptic episodes can be divided into two main forms, absence seizures and major epilepsy. Let's look at absence seizures first.

Absence Seizures

Background information
Absence seizures may not even be noticed by the person with First Aid knowledge unless he knows the casualty well. Even then he may put the episode down to day-dreaming.

Recognition features

✗ *The casualty may appear to stare blankly*

✗ *There may be slight twitching movements*

✗ *There may be strange automatic movements such as lip smacking, chewing, making odd noises, etc*

Aim
● *Protect the casualty until fully recovered*

Actions

1 Help the casualty to sit down in a safe place, privately if possible.

2 Talk to him, and reassure him. Do not ask him questions until he is fully recovered.

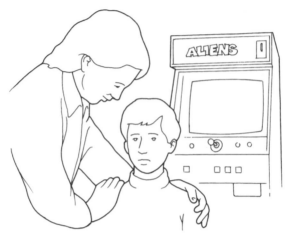

3 If a casualty says that he has not suffered from this condition before then strongly advise him to see his doctor.

Major Epilepsy

Background Information

Major epilepsy is more of a problem for the person with First Aid knowledge.

In this form of the condition the casualty will lose consciousness, collapse and suffer from a seizure.

Recognition features

X *The casualty may notice a strange taste or smell or be aware of the impending episode*

X *Sudden loss of consciousness*

X *The casualty will collapse, sometimes letting out a cry*

X *The body becomes rigid and the back may arch*

X *Breathing may cease and the casualty will develop a blueness to the lips*

X *The face may appear congested*

X *The casualty then starts a series of convulsive movements*

X *The jaw may be clenched and saliva appear at the mouth. This may be blood stained*

X *The casualty may lose control of her bladder and bowels*

X *After a minute or so the casualty becomes relaxed*

X *When the casualty regains consciousness she may be confused for a short period*

X *The casualty may want to sleep following a seizure*

Aims

● *Protect the person from injury during the seizure*

● *Provide care for the person when they regain consciousness*

Actions

1 Try to protect the casualty by removing danger from around them, only move the casualty from danger if there is no other option.

2 Try to protect the head with a cushion or coat.

3 Loosen clothing around the neck.

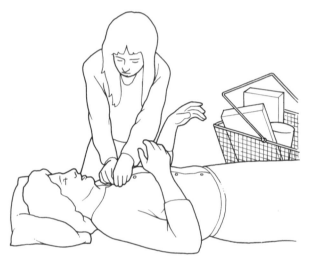

4 Do not try to put anything in the mouth.

5 When the seizure has finished place the person in the recovery position.

In most cases the casualty will not need to go to hospital but would appreciate somewhere private to compose themselves. But, you will need to call an ambulance if:

● **The seizures are repeated.**

● **The casualty is unconscious for more than 10 minutes.**

● **It is the first seizure that the person has had or they sustain an injury during the episode requiring hospital treatment.**

Recognition and Treatment of a Stroke

Background Information

A stroke occurs when a portion of the brain is starved of oxygen due to a burst blood vessel or a clot blocking a blood vessel. This starving of oxygen will cause damage to the brain. The long-term effects are dependent on where the episode occurs in the brain, and how much tissue is affected.

Recognition features

✗ Sudden and severe headache

✗ Confusion, emotional instability

✗ A deterioration in the level of consciousness (this may be sudden or progressive)

✗ Signs of weakness or paralysis usually affecting one side of the body

✗ Slurring or loss of speech

✗ Unequal pupils

✗ Possible loss of bladder and bowel control

Aims

● Maintain the casualty's airway

● Minimise brain damage

● Get urgent medical aid

Actions

1. If the casualty is conscious lay him down, keeping the head and shoulders raised and turn the head to one side if he is dribbling.

2 Place an absorbent pad under the chin if he is dribbling.

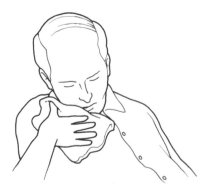

3 Loosen any tight clothing.

4 Talk gently and calmly to the casualty, remember that you may not understand the casualty's replies.

5 Do not give anything to eat or drink.

6 If he is unconscious, then place in the recovery position and maintain a close check on the airway.

7 Dial 999 for an ambulance.

8 Be prepared to resuscitate.

The General Treatment of Poisoning

Background Information

A poison is a substance that when taken into the body in a high enough quantity will cause harm or death. It is beyond the scope of this publication to list and describe the recognition features of all the common poisons that the person with First Aid knowledge may come across. What can be dealt with in this book are general guidelines for dealing with poisons depending on how they have entered the body.

Most episodes of poisoning occur with young children in the home and simple prevention can stop these tragedies:

● Keep dangerous chemicals out of reach

● Keep medicines in a locked cupboard

● Do not transfer substances from one container to another, especially old soft drinks bottles

● Buy all medicines and household substances in child-proof containers

Aims

● *Maintenance of an open airway, breathing and circulation*

● *Maintain or make safe an environment for the casualty and yourself*

● *To obtain urgent medical aid*

● *To identify the poison if possible*

Inhaled poisons

Actions

1 Remove the casualty to open air or open windows without endangering yourself.

2 If possible cut off the source of the poison.

3 Make your initial assessment.

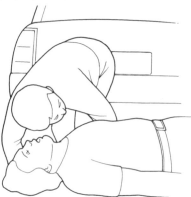

4 If the casualty is breathing but unconscious, place in the recovery position and monitor breathing constantly.

5 If the casualty has stopped breathing, commence artificial ventilation and chest compressions, if required.

6 Contact the emergency services.

Swallowed Poisons

Actions

1 Conduct a primary survey.

2 If the casualty is unconscious and breathing then place in the recovery position, monitor and be prepared to resuscitate.

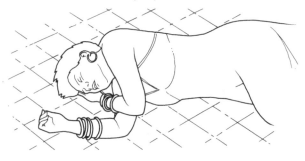

3 If the casualty is conscious, place in a comfortable position and attempt to find out what has been taken. *Do not try to induce vomiting.*

4 If the casualty has taken a corrosive poison then give frequent sips of water, or milk if water is unavailable. If the casualty needs resuscitation then you will need to use a barrier to protect yourself. A polythene bag with a hole punched in for the mouth will suffice in an emergency. "Face Shields" can be obtained from St. John Ambulance for use in an emergency.

5 If the casualty vomits, save a specimen for the emergency services.

6 If possible identify the container(s) that held the poison and save for the emergency services.

Skin Contact

Actions

1 Do not touch the affected area with your bare hands.

2 Flush away any residual poison with copious amounts of running water. Avoid splashing onto yourself or into the casualty's eyes, mouth and nose. If the chemical is causing burns then you will need to keep up the flushing for at least 20 minutes.

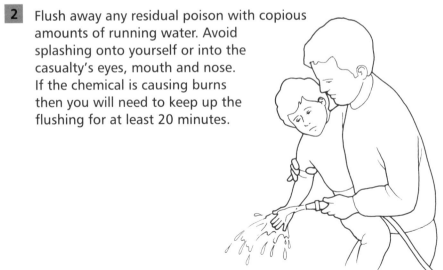

3 Remove any clothing contaminated by the poison where possible and if safe to do so. Try to preserve the casualty's privacy and modesty if possible.

4 If the casualty is unconscious then place into the recovery position and monitor breathing constantly. Be prepared to resuscitate.
If the face is contaminated then you will need to use a barrier.
(See previous page).

Injected Poisons

Actions

1 If the casualty is unconscious and breathing then place in the recovery position and monitor breathing constantly. Be prepared to resuscitate.

2 If the casualty is conscious, place in a comfortable position; keep them as calm and quiet as possible. Monitor the levels of response, breathing and pulse.

3 If possible identify the injected substance. Keep any syringes, needles or samples of the substance etc. for the emergency services. Be extremely careful when dealing with syringes, etc. as these may be contaminated with blood.

The Treatment of Bites and Stings

Background Information

Bites and stings can be painful and distressing injuries, especially to children. Thankfully in the United Kingdom there are no native animals or insects that have a bite or sting that can be classed as highly poisonous. But people do keep such animals as pets and these occasionally cause a problem. We do, however, have a significant number of creatures that can cause a painful bite or sting that may cause localised damage if not dealt with properly.

The person with First Aid knowledge must also remember that a proportion of the population will also suffer a massive allergic reaction to stings. This is known as "Anaphylactic Shock".

Anaphylactic Shock

Background Information

This is a severe allergic reaction that can occur within seconds when stung or bitten by an insect. It may also occur if a person takes a drug that they are allergic to or if they eat a food known to cause a reaction. The main problem that the casualty will suffer is breathing difficulties, which is not only very frightening, but also life threatening.

Recognition Features

X *Anxiety*

X *Widespread blotchy red rash*

X *Swelling of the face and neck*

X *Difficulty with breathing (similar to asthma)*

X *Rapid pulse*

Aim

● *Obtain urgent medical aid*

Actions

1 Dial 999 for an ambulance.

2 Find out if the casualty is carrying any necessary medication (eg. epinephrine in either a syringe or auto-injecter). If necessary, help them to use it.

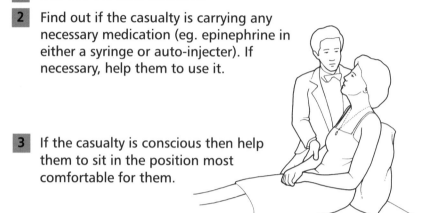

3 If the casualty is conscious then help them to sit in the position most comfortable for them.

4 Reassure them, and monitor closely.

5 If the casualty is unconscious and breathing place in the recovery position, monitor breathing constantly and be prepared to resuscitate.

Animal Bites

Background Information

When an animal bites, it causes two types of wound:

● Superficial lacerations involving crushing and bruising of tissue

● Deep puncture wounds

The puncture wound will cause the greater problem for the casualty as germs will be injected deep into the wound.

Aims

● *To control bleeding*

● *To minimise the risk of infection to yourself and the casualty*

● *To obtain medical attention*

Actions

1 For superficial wounds flush with running water for at least five minutes.

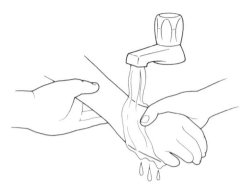

2 Wash the wound, using soap and water.

3 When dry, cover with a sterile dressing.

4 Advise the casualty to seek medical advice and to check whether an anti-tetanus injection is required.

5 For more serious wounds, control the bleeding with direct pressure.

6 Cover with a sterile dressing and take or send the casualty to hospital.

Insect Stings

Background Information

Insect stings on the whole are painful but, unless the casualty is allergic to them, the sting occurs in the mouth, or there are multiple stings, there should be no complications.

Aims

- *To relieve pain and swelling*
- *To obtain medical aid if required*

Actions

1 If visible, carefully remove the sting by gently scraping it off. Take care not to squeeze any poison sac attached.

2 Apply a cold compress to relieve pain and swelling.

3 Advise the casualty to see her own doctor if the pain and swelling do not reduce over the next day or so.

4 If the sting occurs in the mouth, encourage the casualty to suck ice or sip cold water, dial 999 for an ambulance, and monitor closely while waiting for help to arrive.

5 If the casualty is a victim of a swarm attack, causing multiple stings, do not approach until it is safe to do so.

6 Place the casualty in the most comfortable position.

7 Keep the casualty quiet, provide reassurance.

8 Dial 999 for an ambulance urgently.

Marine Stings and Puncture Wounds

Background Information

Sea creatures cause injury in two ways:

- Stinging cells from creatures such as jelly fish and anemone
- Venom spines from urchins or weaver fish, for example

In the UK these cause very painful wounds with localised damage. However, in other parts of the world there are marine creatures that may give a potentially fatal sting.

Marine Stings

Aims

- *To reassure the casualty*
- *To deactivate any remaining cells*
- *To neutralise any free venom*
- *To relieve pain and discomfort*

Actions

1 Hold an ice pack or cold compress against the skin for 10 minutes to relieve pain and swelling. Raise the affected part.

2 In the case of tropical jellyfish, pour seawater or vinegar over the injury to incapacitate the stinging cells. Lightly compress the limb above the sting with a roller bandage, and immobilise the injured limb.

3 If the injury is severe or extensive then arrange an ambulance to take the casualty to hospital.

Marine Puncture Wounds

Aims

- **To deactivate the venom**
- **To obtain medical aid**

1

Actions

Place the injury into as hot water as the casualty can bear without scalding occurring. The injury will need to stay in hot water for at least 30 minutes. Keep the water topped up but be careful not to scald the casualty.

2

Arrange transport for the casualty to go to hospital to have the spines removed.

Snake Bites

Background Information

There is only one poisonous snake in the UK, the adder, but its bite is rarely fatal. However, the casualty can deteriorate through fear rather than the venom. In other countries this can be a different picture with some extremely venomous snakes causing fatalities every year. The person with First Aid knowledge must also remember that some people keep venomous snakes as pets. If you suspect that you are dealing with a bite from a snake then try to get a description of the snake and inform the police.

Aims

- *To reassure the casualty*
- *To prevent the spread of venom*
- *To obtain urgent medical aid*

1 Lay the casualty down and explain to them the importance of remaining calm.

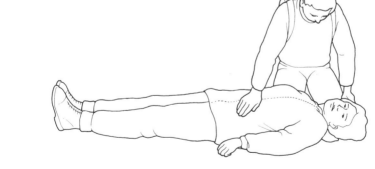

2 Wash the wound with soap and water, if available. Do not try to suck or cut venom from the wound and do not apply a tourniquet.

3 Secure and support the injured limb.

4 Monitor the casualty's consciousness, breathing and pulse.

5 Dial 999 for an ambulance.

What Next?

This book has provided you with the guidance that you need to give Emergency Aid. It is, however, no substitute for a proper First Aid course. Rescue Breaths and CPR must be practised under qualified supervision.

Please, then, consider taking a St. John course. The following are offered in all Counties in England and Wales.

First Aid at Work course (24 hours' instruction)
This is a course which leads to the statutory certificate recognised by the Health and Safety Executive. It is additionally a useful extra qualification for school leavers as it is valued by employers who, by law, have to provide qualified First Aiders on their premises.

Emergency Aid courses (4 hours' instruction)
These are short introductory courses containing a wide range of information. They can be modified to meet the needs of the general public or the Appointed Person in the work place.

Lifesaver First Aid courses
St. John Ambulance has introduced a new range of courses which involve the student more in the learning process. The courses form a programme and you can decide which parts of the programme are relevant to you. These courses are designed to enable you to be confident and competent in the skills at the end of the course.

The courses include:

Lifesaver First Aid course (8 hours)
This course covers the basic lifesaving techniques for an adult.

Lifesaver Plus course (8 hours + 2 hours' optional examination)
This course follows on from the Lifesaver course and builds on it by adding information on a wide range of injuries and conditions.

Lifesaver for Babies and Children (4 hours)
This course stands alone and deals with the lifesaving techniques for babies and children.

Details of all St. John courses are available from your County Headquarters. Call your nearest Headquarters on 08700 10 49 50 or contact: St. John Ambulance National Headquarters, 27 St. John's Lane, London EC1M 4BU. Tel: 020 7324 4000 Fax: 020 7324 4001

First Aid Supplies
St. John Supplies offer a range of products including First Aid kits, books and videos. All profits from the sale of these go to support the work of St. John Ambulance. For further details or a catalogue, please contact:
St. John Supplies, PO Box 707B, Friend Street, London EC1V 7NE
Tel: 020 7278 7888 Fax: 020 7278 1642